YOUR KNOWLEDGE HAS VALUE

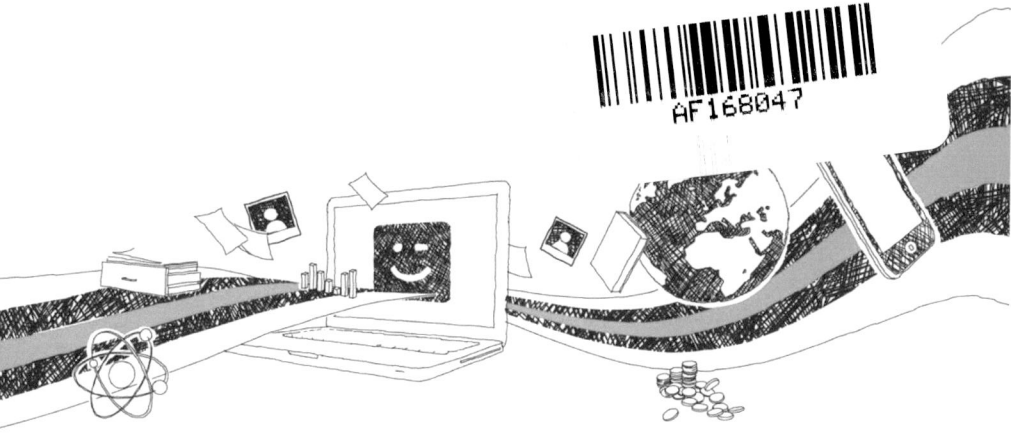

- We will publish your bachelor's and master's thesis, essays and papers

- Your own eBook and book - sold worldwide in all relevant shops

- Earn money with each sale

Upload your text at www.GRIN.com
and publish for free

Bibliographic information published by the German National Library:

The German National Library lists this publication in the National Bibliography; detailed bibliographic data are available on the Internet at http://dnb.dnb.de .

Imprint:

Copyright © 2020 GRIN Verlag
Print and binding: Books on Demand GmbH, Norderstedt Germany
ISBN: 9783346206176

This book at GRIN:

https://www.grin.com/document/903760

Samuel Lehmann

Social Determinants of Health Impacting Young Adults aged 18 to 25. Stress and Addiction

GRIN Verlag

GRIN - Your knowledge has value

Since its foundation in 1998, GRIN has specialized in publishing academic texts by students, college teachers and other academics as e-book and printed book. The website www.grin.com is an ideal platform for presenting term papers, final papers, scientific essays, dissertations and specialist books.

Visit us on the internet:

http://www.grin.com/

http://www.facebook.com/grincom

http://www.twitter.com/grin_com

Social Determinants of Health Impacting Young Adults aged 18-25: Stress and Addiction

University: James Cook University

College: College of Healthcare Sciences

Health Promotion for Health Professionals

Student Name: Samuel Lehmann

Table of Contents

Despite the importance of medical care itself, public health is becoming increasingly aware of, and vigilant in addressing, the social and economic conditions that predispose the public to poor health in the first place (Wilkinson, & Marmot, 2003). The identified sensitivity of human health to the broader social environment has given rise to the proposed 10 social determinants of health (SDoH) (AIHW, 2016). These include social gradient, stress, early life, social exclusion, working conditions, unemployment, social support, addiction, food and transport (Wilkinson, & Marmot, 2003). Their importance lies in the potential development of public policy frameworks, targeting each determinant and facilitating the overcoming of socioeconomic barriers to achieve improved health outcomes (AIHW, 2016). Accordingly, the following report aims to outline the influence of two SDoH, stress and addiction, among the young adult (YA) population (18-25 years). The implications of the SDoH on providing care as a physiotherapist will also be discussed and evaluated at both the individual and broader community levels.

Stress

Stress is a term encompassing various forms and can stem from multiple aspects of individuals' lives. It refers to the influence of factors such as perceived demand from an individual's environment, a response to a threatening situation and external stressors including life events, relationships and work (Bovier et al., 2004). Generally, stress induces long-term health effects, such as constant release of stress hormones, raised heart rate and blood pressure and diverting blood away from many physiological processes vital to health-maintenance (Wilkinson, & Marmot, 2003).

More specifically, YAs have been identified as susceptible and likely to experience stress during the transitionary phase from school to either tertiary education or directly to the workforce (Zunhammer et al., 2014). Pascoe et al. (2019) highlighted that across 77 countries, 66% and 59% of tertiary students reported feeling stressed regarding poor examination results and difficulty of upcoming tests, respectively. This prevalence among university students is especially relevant when considering that 59% of Australian school leavers enrol in tertiary study (ABS, 2019). For the 29% of Australian school leavers entering the workforce, stress also arises as a significant health risk factor (ABS, 2019). Sawang and Newton (2018) interviewed 18 young Australian workers, uncovering that stress emerges in YAs' working lives most commonly due to perceived incompetence damaging self-esteem, interpersonal conflict and belittlement from older colleagues.

The implications of stress on YAs are vast and significant throughout the social, mental and physical domains of their lives (Sawang & Newton, 2018). Stress is undoubtably associated with mental health; in particular anxiety and depression have proven to be eventual by-products of high stress levels (Pascoe et al., 2019). Accordingly, Pascoe et al. (2019) documented that academic-related stress in university students has led to 35% and 30% of tertiary students experiencing anxiety and depression, respectively. The repercussions of this are clear in the findings that examination performance is hindered in students dealing with stress, anxiety and depression, resulting in a vicious circle as poor results further impact students' mental health (Pascoe et al., 2019).

From a physical health perspective, research conducted by Zunhammer et al. (2013) reinforced the presence of a spike in stress, anxiety and depression in students surrounding examinations. Alarmingly, students commonly reported stress-related symptoms such as nausea, diarrhea, loss of appetite and gastro-intestinal pain leading up to and during examination periods (Zunhammer et al., 2013). Furthermore, Zunhammer at al., (2013) revealed that students are prone to suffering from insomnia during examination periods, according to the identified half-hour average decrease in daily sleep. The reported decreases in sleep time was attributed to cognitive mechanisms such as hyperarousal and rumination occurring in response to examination stress (Zunhammer at al., 2013). Sexual health is also influenced by stress, as Dimou et al. (2013) discovered that increased levels of stress in YAs strongly correlated with unsafe sexual practices, decreased testosterone levels in males and menstrual cycle disturbances in females.

4

Clearly, academic and work-related stress serve as threats to the health of YAs, both psychosocially and physically. In response to this, interventions must be sought and implemented to reduce the impact of stress in YAs. For instance, a study examining the relationship between stress and sexual health in YAs involved the administering of twice-daily, evidence-based guided relaxation over a period of eight weeks; proving effective in reducing stress and subsequently improving sexual health (Dimou et al., 2013).

Addiction

Circumstances involving an individual presenting with cravings, impaired self-control and development of tolerance and withdrawal symptoms, resembles addiction associated with an aspect of their life (Thomée et al., 2011). Addictions commonly arise as they may offer an escape from adversities and external stressors; and are pertinent to the lives and health of many YAs (Wilkinson & Marmot, 2003). The debilitating short and long-term impacts of addiction on quality of life are undeniable, exacerbated by its tendency to overlap, interconnecting various addiction types (Wilkinson & Marmot, 2003).

Mobile phone and social media dependence among YAs is considered a form of addiction, with research identifying corresponding symptoms of withdrawal, separation anxiety and impaired self-control in young Australian adults (Lyvers et al., 2018). Its prevalence is certainly widespread as an estimated 32% of young Australian adults spend at least two hours on social media daily (Lyvers et al., 2018). Additionally, studies have revealed an increasing relationship between mobile phone dependence and level of education as university students displayed greater symptom levels, further proving the prevalence of social media addiction in YAs (Oviedo-Trespalacios et al., 2019).

Furthermore, alcohol consumption has been identified as another widespread addiction carrying significant health implications throughout the YA population (Mewton et al., 2011). McKenzie et al. (2011) reported that 19% of YAs in Australia were diagnosed with an alcohol use disorder (AUD), with approximately 60% of this subset consuming at least five

5

standard drinks, on average, once each week. The predisposition of YAs to alcohol addiction presents itself due to their newfound financial and social independence encountered as they leave school and begin working or studying full-time (McKenzie et al., 2011). Moreover, McKenzie et al., (2011) discovered an association between depression and anxiety experienced as a teenager, and AUD diagnosis as a YA. It was found that AUD prevalence in those who experienced more than two waves of moderate to severe adolescent depression and anxiety symptoms (27%) greatly exceeded those who experienced few symptoms (17%), establishing the crucial link between stress, poor mental health and alcohol addiction (McKenzie et al., 2011).

As a consequence of widespread alcohol and social media addiction, YAs are evidently more susceptible to poor mental and physical health outcomes (Mewton et al., 2011). Mobile phone dependence was shown in multiple studies to both trigger and amplify symptoms of anxiety, depression and insomnia in YAs (Thomée et al., 2011). Similarly, 60% of YAs diagnosed with an AUD were also diagnosed with at least one mental health disorder and 8% reported suicidal thoughts, behaviours or attempts (Mewton et al., 2011). In addition, long-term physical health implications such as cancer, dementia and liver disease, along with the short-term risks including traffic accidents, unsafe sex and violence, substantiate the threat posed by alcohol to YAs (Mewton et al., 2011).

Combined, the works of Lyvers et al., (2018) and Mewton et al., (2011) established a connection between mobile phone and alcohol addictions in YAs as long-term predictors of illicit substance addiction. These findings were attributed to congruencies in the criteria commonly met for each addiction; including rash impulsivity and narcissism, along with the fact that YAs diagnosed with an AUD were 15 times more likely to have an illicit drug addiction (Lyvers et al., 2018; Mewton et al., 2011). Accordingly, it is absolutely pivotal that health professionals consider interventions combatting impulsive behaviour, anxiety and depression during adolescence in order to prevent mobile phone, alcohol and drug addictions in YAs (Lyvers et al., 2018).

The SDoH are embedded in health promotion strategies as they directly influence the prevalence of health inequity; the avoidable, systemic differences in health status across socioeconomic groups (Paz, 2012). Health promotion is a concept unpinning the Ottawa Charter, a framework encompassing the advocation, enablement and mediation of people to gain control over the improvement of their health (Fry & Zask, 2017). It aims to achieve this across five key action areas; developing personal skills, strengthening community action, creating supportive environments, building healthy public policy and reorientating health services (Fry & Zask, 2017). In doing so, the Ottawa Charter widens the scope of public health beyond individual behaviours and risk factors to also consider the socioeconomic factors influencing health outcomes across populations (Fish & Moffatt, 2014). Accordingly, physiotherapists are able to effectively ensure positive health outcomes across populations by utilising health promotion strategies, as outlined by the Ottawa Charter, at both individual and community levels.

Individual

The Ottawa Charter describes downstream health promotion strategies as those that target the immediate health needs of individuals, while seeking to increase equitable access to health and social services (Fish & Moffatt, 2014). This constitutes the basis of physiotherapy, involving the use of physical approaches that aim to restore, maintain and promote physical, social and psychological well-being (Boakye et al., 2018). As a physiotherapist, it is imperative to investigate the socioeconomic factors contributing to patients' health outcomes in order to ensure that the treatment, as well as implemented maintenance and prevention strategies, are suitable and sustainable (Bezner, 2015).

Developing personal skills and reorientating health services are two key action areas, as addressed by the Ottawa Charter, applicable to physiotherapists when considering SDoH in their provision of care (Fry & Zask, 2017). For example, a patient's unemployment status may be attributed to an injury sustained due to suboptimal working conditions, such as strenuous manual labour or extensive sedentary periods (Yasobant & Mohanty, 2017). A physiotherapist can then intervene using rehabilitation to return the individual to work and implement prevention strategies addressing the original cause. Furthermore, the implementation of home physiotherapy services can eliminate the barrier often posed by transport and social gradient to individuals who are logistically or financially unable to travel to a primary health care setting (Paz, 2012). On another note, compliance to physiotherapy treatment and rehabilitation is largely determined by an individual's exposure to social support. If a lack of social support for an individual is identified, motivational interviewing can be employed by physiotherapists to increase a patient's motivation to improve health behaviours (Bezner, 2015).

However, the effectiveness of health promotion strategies cannot be unlocked if social determinant screening isn't performed. Yasobant and Mohanty, (2017) discovered that physiotherapists reported time constraints and the focus of acute settings on discharge as the main perceived barriers to performing screening. Hence, mitigation of these barriers should be prioritised in order to ensure effective consideration of SDoH in physiotherapy.

Community

Physiotherapists can also employ health promotion strategies using an upstream approach, targeting factors such as social status, income, exclusion and living conditions by building healthy public policy, strengthening community action and creating supportive environments (Fry & Zask, 2017). In doing so, interventions, programs and policies can be implemented or adapted to improve health outcomes across communities. Interventions such as community-based fall prevention programs for seniors are a means to improve health outcomes while reducing the prevalence of social exclusion among elderly individuals (Yasobant & Mohanty, 2017). Moreover, in communities where elderly residents report feeling unsafe exercising outside, group intervention is especially applicable (Rethorn, 2018). Rethorn (2018) identified this as a physiotherapist and responded by leading walks with groups of patients, effectively improving their perception of safety in their neighbourhood.

In terms of policies, there are many avenues physiotherapists can take to structurally improve health outcomes. In cases where poor working conditions may lead to musculoskeletal injury, such as strenuous manual labour or prolonged sedentary periods, physiotherapists can work with companies and organisations to implement policies containing injury prevention measures (Yasobant & Mohanty, 2017). These could include the introduction of signs displaying correct lifting techniques, limits placed on maximum lifting amounts or ergonomic improvements to desk arrangements in office settings; each strategy aiming to manage injury at its source (Yasobant & Mohanty, 2017). Physiotherapists can also collaborate with town planners to ensure public spaces are designed to support the physical activity needs of the community across all ability levels (Bezner, 2015). Health education, such as education of school students on the importance of diet and physical activity in preventing obesity and comorbidities, currently serves as the most commonly utilised health promotion strategy by physiotherapists (Mokwena & Phetlhe, 2015). However, the importance of community intervention and policy implementation is evident and must be further foregrounded.

Conclusion

When considering the identified impacts of stress and addiction on the health of YAs, the association between the SDoH and health outcomes across populations is irrefutable. It was revealed that various forms of stress and addiction carry the potential to detrimentally influence mental and sexual health, sleep and even predisposition to the development of substance addiction in YAs. The relevance of the SDoH to physiotherapy practice was also explored with reference to the Ottawa Charter. A range of suitable health promotion strategies were outlined with the intent of improving health outcomes at both the individual and community levels via downstream and upstream intervention approaches, respectively.

References

ABS. (2019). *Education and Work, Australia, May 2019* (No. 6227.0).
https://www.abs.gov.au/ausstats%5Cabs@.nsf/mediareleasesbyCatalogue/D422D01
60CA82AE8CA25750C00117DD1

AIHW. (2016). *Australia's health 2016* (No. 199).
https://www.aihw.gov.au/reports/australias-health/australias-health-
2016/contents/determinants

Bezner, J. R. (2015). Promoting Health and Wellness: Implications for Physical Therapist
Practice. *Physical Therapy, 95*(10), 1433-1444. https://doi.org/10.2522/ptj.20140271

Boakye, H., Quartey, J., Baidoo, N. A. B., & Ahenkorah, J. (2018). Knowledge, attitude and
practice of physiotherapists towards health promotion in Ghana. *South African
Journal of Physiotherapy, 74*(1), 443. https://doi.org/10.4102/sajp.v74i1.443

Bovier, P. A., Chamot, E., Perneger, T. V. (2004). Perceived Stress, Internal Resources, and
Social Support as Determinants of Mental Health among Young Adults. *Quality of Life
Research, 13*(1), 161,170. https://doi.org/10.1023/B:QURE.0000015288.43768.e4

Dimou, P. A., Bacopoulou, F., Darviri, C., & Chrousos, G.P. (2013). Stress management and
sexual health of young adults: a pilot randomised controlled trial. *First International
Journal of Andrology, 46*(9), 1022-1031. https://doi.org/10.1111/and.12190

Fish, K., & Moffatt, H. (2014). National Collaborating Centre for Determinants of Health.
Let's talk: Moving upstream. Antigonish, NS: National Collaborating Centre for
Determinants of Health, St. Francis Xavier University.

Fry, D., & Zask, A. (2017). Applying the Ottawa Charter to inform health promotion
programme design. *Health Promotion International, 32*(5), 901-912.
https://doi.org/10.1093/heapro/daw022

Lyvers, M., Narayanan, S. S., & Thorberg, F. A. (2018). Disordered social media use and risky
drinking in young adults: Differential associations with addiction-linked traits.
Australian Journal of Psychology, 71(3), 223-231. https://doi.org/10.1111/ajpy.12236

McKenzie, M., Jorm, A. F., Romaniuk, H., Olsson, C. A., & Patton, G. C. (2011). Association of adolescent symptoms of depression and anxiety with alcohol use disorders in young adulthood: findings from the Victorian Adolescent Health Cohort Study. *Med J Aust, 195*(3). https://doi.org/10.5694/j.1326-5377.2011.tb03262.x

Mewton, L., Teesson, M., Slade, T., & Grove, R. (2011). The Epidemiology of DSM-IV Alcohol Use Disorders amongst Young Adults in the Australian Population. *Alcohol and Alcoholism, 46*(2), 185-191. https://doi.org/10.1093/alcalc/agq091

Mokwena, K., & Phetlhe, K. (2015). Assessment of health promotion content in undergraduate physiotherapy curricula. *South African Journal of Physiotherapy, 71*(1), 242. https://doi.org/10.4102/sajp.v71i1.242

Oviedo-Trespalacios, O., Nandavar, S., Newton, J. D. A., Demant, D., & Phillips, J. G. (2019). Problematic Use of Mobile Phones in Australia…Is It Getting Worse? *Frontiers in Psychiatry, 10*(105). https://doi.org/10.3389/fpsyt.2019.00105

Pascoe, M. C., Hetrick, S. E., & Parker, A. G. (2019). The impact of stress on students in secondary school and higher education. *International Journal of Adolescence and Youth, 25*(1), 104-112. https://doi.org/10.1080/02673843.2019.1596823

Paz, B. (2012). Home Physiotherapy: The Relevance of Social Determinants of Health in the Development of Physiotherapy in the Home Environment. https://doi.org/10.5772/35275

Pennay, A., Lubman, D. I., & MacLean, S. (2011). Risky drinking among young Australians. *Australian Family Physician, 40*(8). https://www.racgp.org.au/download/documents/AFP/2011/August/201108pennay.pdf

Rethorn, Z. D. (2018). *When Health Decisions Aren't a Matter of Choice: Addressing Social Determinants of Health.* http://www.apta.org/Blogs/PTTransforms/2018/10/10/SocialDeterminants/

Sawang, S., Newton, C. J. (2018). Defining Work Stress in Young People. *Journal of Employment Counseling, 55*(2), 72-83. https://doi.org/10.1002/joec.12076

Thomée, S., Härenstam, A., & Hagberg, M. (2011). Mobile phone use and stress, sleep disturbances, and symptoms of depression among young adults - a prospective cohort study. *BMC Public Health, 11*(66). https://doi.org/10.1186/1471-2458-11-66

Wilkinson, R, & Marmot, M. (Ed.). (2003). *Social determinants of health: The solid facts.* http://www.euro.who.int/__data/assets/pdf_file/0005/98438/e81384.pdf

Yasobant, S. Mohanty, S. (2017). Would Physiotherapists be Public Health Promoters?: Concern or Opportunity for Indian Public Health System. *Austin Journal of Palliative Care, 2*(1). https://www.researchgate.net/publication/316033865_Would_Physiotherapists_be_Public_Health_Promoters_Concern_or_Opportunity_for_Indian_Public_Health_System

Zunhammer, M., Eberle, H., Eichhammer, P., & Busch, V. (2013). Somatic Symptoms Evoked by Exam Stress in University Students: The Role of Alexithymia, Neuroticism, Anxiety and Depression. *PLoS One, 8*(12). https://doi.org/10.1371/journal.pone.0084911

Zunhammer, M., Eichhammer, P., & Busch, V. (2014). Sleep Quality during Exam Stress: The Role of Alcohol, Caffeine and Nicotine. *PLoS One, 9*(10). https://doi.org/10.1371/journal.pone.0109490

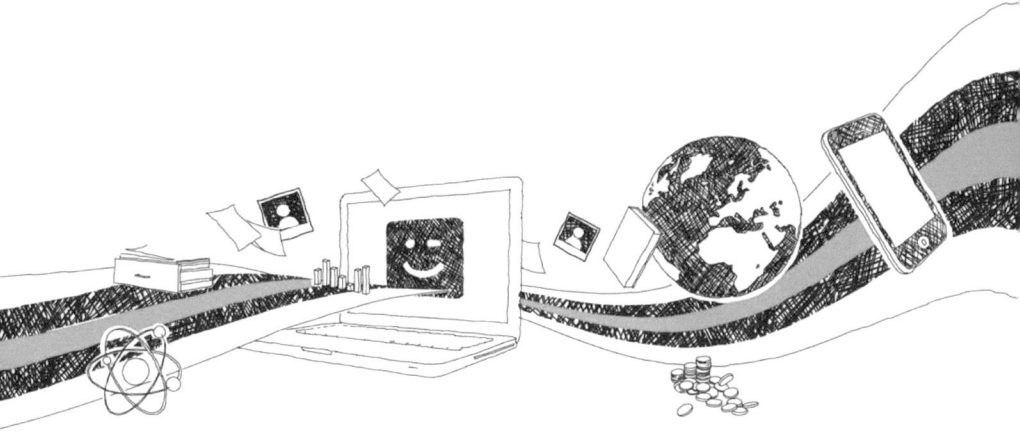
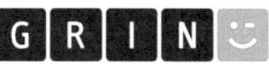